PAXLOVID FOR BEGINNERS

The Dependable Guide Used in Adults to Treat Mild to Moderate Coronavirus and Omicron in Patients who have a Positive Result from SARS-CoV-2 Viral Test

Nathan Mccalister
Copyright@2022

D0095610

TABLE OF CONTENT

CHAPTER 1
OUTLINE

In July, Joe Biden, the Vice President of the United States, was given the antiviral medicine Paxlovid after a test revealed that he was infected with the Covid-19 virus. If highly sensitive individuals who get infected with Covid use this prescription drug outside of a hospital environment, they may be able to avoid the development of severe symptoms, including some that might prove deadly.

Paxlovid is the first oral Covid antiviral to be made accessible to patients after receiving approval from both the Food and Drug Administration (FDA) and the UK Medicines and Healthcare Products Regulatory Agency (UK Medicines and Healthcare Products Regulatory Agency) in December 2021. Because of the lightning-fast rate at which it was authorized by authorities less than a year after the first patient obtained the treatment in clinical trials, it has been labeled the shortest drug-development project in

4

the history of the industry. This distinction was bestowed upon it.

Since then, the European Medicines Agency has granted approval for Paxlovid, and the United Nations has begun negotiations with pharmaceutical companies to begin production of a generic version of the drug in April 2022. At that time, millions of pills will be distributed to countries that have low or middle incomes.

CHAPTER 2

The Role That Paxlovid Plays in the Body

Both nirmatrelvir and ritonavir are components of the combination therapy known as Paxlovid, which was developed by the multinational pharmaceutical corporation Pfizer.

Once the SARS-CoV-2 virus has entered a cell, it will utilize its own machinery to make the proteins that it requires in order to produce new copies of itself. This will enable the virus to continue to spread.

Nirmatrelvir, an antiviral component of Paxlovid, is the factor that contributes to the medication's efficacy. It does this by blocking an enzyme known as Mpro, which is found in many different coronaviruses and is responsible for the replication of coronaviruses. Nirmatrelvir is capable of inhibiting the capacity of Mpro to create the functional proteins that are essential for

7

the replication of SARS-CoV-2. Pfizer developed it in 2002 in response to the first epidemic of SARS, thus it has some background in the fight against the disease.

Another drug called ritonavir is used as a "boosting agent" in treatment. The metabolism of nirmatrelvir is delayed, which results in higher concentrations of the active antiviral and a longer half-life in the body. In the past, ritonavir was used to enhance the effectiveness of HIV antiviral therapy.

CHAPTER 3

How do you take Paxlovid?

When using Paxlovid, patients are instructed to take two tablets of nirmatrelvir (each containing 50 milligrams) and one pill of ritonavir (containing 100 milligrams) twice daily for a period of five days. Paxlovid should be administered as soon as feasible after infection, and at the very latest during the first five days following the beginning of symptoms, in order to prevent the development of full-blown

Covid. This should be done as soon as possible.

In what ways does it accomplish its goals?

Paxlovid is now the most popular choice among oral antivirals available for the treatment of Covid. In order to get permission from the relevant authorities, a clinical research had to be carried out, and the findings revealed that patients treated with Covid had an 89 percent lower chance of hospitalization and fatality.

It has been shown to be beneficial in really terrible conditions, but in less catastrophic circumstances, its use is less clear. In a study that was carried out by Pfizer, there was not a significant enough difference in the outcomes of those who had taken Paxlovid and those who had not taken the medication for the researchers to draw the conclusion that the treatment was effective in preventing infections in people who had been exposed to a

12

symptomatic household contact within the previous four days.

In a similar vein, it has not lived up to the hopes that it would be beneficial in the treatment of those who are suffering from very mild illnesses. Paxlovid's effects on patients with standard-risk Covid were evaluated in a research that was conducted in June. Because the patients' symptoms did not meaningfully improve, the study was terminated.

Paxlovid is not used to prevent the development of symptoms or to prevent infection after exposure; nevertheless, it is helpful in preventing the most severe symptoms of Covid in those who are at high risk for the illness.

CHAPTER 4

Does it also have an effect on the More Recent Variants?

It would seem such is the situation. Nirmatrelvir was shown to decrease Mpro activity in the wild-type SARS-CoV-2 virus as well as in the virus's Alpha, Beta, Delta, Gamma, and Omicron subtypes, according to an announcement made by Pfizer in February 2022.

Researchers from the University of Tokyo have shown, using grown monkey cells, that the antiviral medication nirmatrelvir is able to stop the transmission of the BA.5 subvariant of Omicron virus. This virus is responsible for the recent outbreak of diseases.

Who Is Allowed Entry?

People in the United Kingdom and the United States who are over the age of 12 and weigh more than 40 kilograms (88 pounds) and who are considered to be at high risk of having severe symptoms, being admitted to the hospital, or dying if they get Covid are eligible to take Paxlovid. In the United Kingdom, this means people who are at high risk of having severe symptoms, being admitted to the hospital, or dying. On the other hand, they must only be having mild or moderate Covid symptoms and cannot have been hospitalized for their current condition at any point in time.

People who are over the age of 65 and people who have certain preexisting conditions, such as HIV, chronic renal disease, numerous autoimmune disorders, Down syndrome, sickle cell disease, some kinds of cancer, and diabetes, are regarded to be at a high risk from Covid. Patients who have already undergone organ transplantation are also regarded as high-risk patients.

CHAPTER 5

Does Paxlovid Have Some Kind of Sign-In Procedure?

The answer to this question will depend on where you now reside. Talk to your healthcare provider if you feel that Paxlovid might be the correct treatment option for you and you have tested positive for HIV in the United States. You also have the option of going to a facility that offers a test called "Test-to-Treat." Here, a pharmacist who is licensed in your state will evaluate your case and decide whether or not you are eligible for the therapy, after which they will provide you with a prescription. Before going to any of these venues, check to see that you have all of the required documentation with you.

You have the option of being tested and submitting your findings online if you reside in the UK, have a suspicion that you have Covid, and satisfy the conditions to be eligible for Paxlovid. If the results of the test show that you are eligible for treatment and they are positive, the NHS will get in touch with you about how to get it. If you feel that you are eligible for NHS services but have not been contacted by the organization, do not be afraid to get in touch with the primary care physician that you see on a regular basis or ring 111.

In the United Kingdom, if you have a prescription for a medication, you have the option of having it delivered to your house or having a friend, member of your family, or volunteer pick it up for you. Patients in the United Kingdom who would normally be eligible for this drug but have been experiencing delays in getting it from the Covid medications distribution site that is closest to them.

CHAPTER 6

What exactly does it imply when someone has a paxlovid rebound?

When a person takes the treatment for Covid and initially exhibits indications of improvement—they test negative—but then, often just a few days later, either they develop symptoms again or they test positive. This happens when a person has a relapse of the condition after taking the medicine for Covid. It would seem that both Vice President Biden and Chief

Medical Advisor to the United States Anthony Fauci were affected by this.

The investigation of the phenomenon is still in its infancy; nonetheless, what is known thus far is that rebound symptoms are frequently mild, and rebounding does not seem to be extremely common. One preliminary study, which is still in preprint form and is waiting for formal review by independent researchers, analyzed the outcomes of

11,000 people who had been treated with Paxlovid and found that 3.5 percent of participants rebounded to test positive again seven days after treatment, with 2.3 percent experiencing the return of symptoms. The study was conducted on people who had been treated with Paxlovid. At 30 days, 5.4% of patients had positive test results again, and 5.9% of patients were having symptoms.

Why does it look like Covid is
making progress again?

Rebounding is not something
that just occurs in people who
are taking Paxlovid; it has also
been seen in patients using
Covid who have not been
treated. Researchers at the
University of California, San
Diego who specialize in
infectious illnesses recently
carried out an exhaustive
research of 568 Covid patients,
and they found that 27% of
those individuals experienced
rebounding symptoms.

It's possible that the mechanism of action behind Paxlovid holds the answer. It is likely that the five-day treatment cycle does not always allow sufficient time for the immune system to get into gear and totally remove the virus. This is because Paxlovid does not really destroy the virus but rather prevents it from growing. After the Paxlovid has been eliminated, there is a possibility that some of the virus that was present during the first infection may begin to replicate once again.

After discontinuing Paxlovid as prescribed, there is a possibility that some people may suffer rebound.

If I have Paxlovid Rebound, are you able to tell me what steps to take?

If you get a positive retest or notice that your Covid symptoms have returned, you need to take steps to lower the risk that you may infect other people with the disease.

If you've gone five days without a fever, you can stop your re-isolation, even if you're still testing positive, but you should still wear a mask for ten days after the onset of rebounding symptoms. For example, in the United States, the Centers for Disease Control and Prevention (CDC) recommends isolating patients for at least five days after the onset of rebounding symptoms. In addition, the CDC recommends isolating patients for at least five days after

29

Will Paxlovid's Efficacy Become Less Effective With Continued Use?

Despite the absence of evidence connecting the two, some experts believe that it is only "a matter of time" until the Paxlovid virus develops resistance to the medication.

In a series of preprints, researchers from KU Leuven, the University of Copenhagen, and Rutgers University demonstrated that the coronavirus is capable of developing resistance to the replication-inhibiting medication nirmatrelvir.

The clinical tests are designed to replicate situations that could occur in real life and in which the virus has a good chance of evolving. These scenarios include an immunocompromised patient who has trouble clearing the virus from their system and an infected individual who does not finish their full course of

Paxlovid. Both of these situations are examples of situations in which the virus has a good chance of evolving.

Researchers have shown that the SARS-CoV-2 virus is capable of replicating even in the presence of nirmatrelvir by accumulating mutations in the amino acid chains that are a component of Mpro.

There is a concern that an increase in the number of prescriptions for Paxlovid will subject the virus to greater selection pressure by providing it with more opportunities to try out changes that might help it survive in the presence of the drug. This raises the possibility that the virus will evolve in a way that makes it more resistant to the effects of the drug.

Even if viruses that are resistant to Paxlovid develop in the future, the medication may still have a role in future treatment strategies if it is combined with other antivirals. This idea should be kept in mind even if it hasn't gotten a lot of attention from people so far.

THE END

Made in the USA
Middletown, DE
30 December 2022